DAILY VAGUS NERVE EXERCISES

Unlock Your Route to Wellness A Comprehensive Guide to Daily Vagus Nerve Stimulation for Reducing Stress, Enhancing Mind-Body Connection, and Igniting Vitality in Just 7 Minutes a Day

Timothy R. Clayton

TABLE OF CONTENTS

Part 1: Introduction to the Vagus Nerve and Its Power

Deep within your body lies a hidden conductor, orchestrating a symphony of vital functions. This maestro is the vagus nerve, the longest cranial nerve in your body, and it holds the key to unlocking a state of deep relaxation, reduced stress, and enhanced well-being.

Chapter 1: Unveiling the Vagus Nerve: Your Body's Mastermind of Calm

Have you ever felt a wave of calm wash over you after a deep breath or a hearty laugh? Thank the vagus nerve! This opening chapter will unveil the fascinating anatomy and function of this powerful nerve.

Demystifying the Vagus Nerve: Anatomy and Function:

Imagine a complex highway system branching out from your brainstem. That's the vagus nerve! We'll explore its intricate path, traveling down your neck, through your chest, and finally reaching your abdomen, influencing organs along the way. You'll learn how it acts as a two-way street, sending messages from your body to your brain and vice versa.

The Vagus Nerve Connection: Stress, Anxiety, and the Path to Wellbeing:

Feeling overwhelmed? The vagus nerve is essential for stress management. When you're stressed, your body activates the "fight-or-flight" response. The vagus nerve acts as a calming counterpoint, promoting relaxation and helping your body return to a balanced state. By stimulating the vagus nerve, you can actively switch off the stress response and promote feelings of peace and well-being.

Chapter 2: Why Daily Vagus Nerve Exercises Matter: Unlocking Your Body's Natural Healing Potential

The vagus nerve isn't just a passive observer in your well-being; it's an active participant with immense potential. This chapter will explore the science behind stimulating the vagus nerve and the many benefits you can reap through daily exercises.

The Science Behind Vagus Nerve Stimulation:

Science is increasingly recognizing the power of the vagus nerve. We'll delve into research that demonstrates how stimulating the vagus nerve can positively impact your mental and physical health. Studies have shown it can:

* Reduce inflammation
* Improve heart rate variability (a marker of stress resilience)
* Enhance mood and emotional regulation

The Benefits of Daily Practice: Reducing Stress, Enhancing Mood, and More:

The benefits of daily vagus nerve exercises extend far beyond simply feeling calmer. Imagine experiencing:

* Reduced stress and anxiety
* Improved digestion and gut health
* Deeper, more restful sleep
* Enhanced emotional regulation and feelings of well-being

These are just a few of the many ways stimulating the vagus nerve can positively impact your life.

By understanding the vagus nerve and its power, you'll be well-equipped to embark on a journey of self-discovery and unlock the potential for a calmer, healthier, and more vibrant you.

Chapter 1: Unveiling the Vagus Nerve: Your Body's Mastermind of Calm

Have you ever wondered what happens inside your body when you take a deep breath and feel a wave of relaxation wash over you? Or perhaps you've experienced a surge of calmness after a hearty laugh. The answer lies within a remarkable nerve called the vagus nerve. Often referred to as the body's "mastermind of calm," the vagus nerve is the longest cranial nerve in your system, and it plays a critical role in promoting relaxation, reducing stress, and influencing a wide range of bodily functions.

- Demystifying the Vagus Nerve: Anatomy and Function

Imagine a complex highway system with a central hub located deep within your brainstem. This hub sends out vital information and receives feedback through a network of interconnected pathways. This elaborate system is precisely what the vagus nerve resembles. Unlike most motor nerves that carry signals only one way (from brain to muscle), the vagus nerve is a mixed nerve. It acts as a two-way street, carrying messages from your brain to various organs throughout your body (motor function) and relaying sensory information back to the brain (sensory function).

The vagus nerve embarks on a fascinating journey. It starts at the base of your brainstem and travels down your neck, branching out through your chest cavity (thorax) and finally reaching your abdomen. Along the way, it sends messages to and receives information from numerous organs, including:

Heart: The vagus nerve helps regulate your heart rate and blood pressure, promoting a slower and steadier beat during times of rest.

Lungs: It plays a role in constricting your airways during coughing and helps regulate your breathing rate.

Digestive System: The vagus nerve significantly influences digestion by stimulating the muscles in your esophagus, stomach, and intestines, ensuring smooth food movement and optimal nutrient absorption.

Other Organs: It also influences functions in the spleen, gallbladder, and even vocal cords.

This intricate network of connections highlights the vagus nerve's vital role in maintaining a state of homeostasis, the balanced internal environment necessary for optimal body function.

- The Vagus Nerve Connection: Stress, Anxiety, and the Path to Wellbeing

Many people in today's fast-paced society live with worry and anxiety all the time. But what if there was a natural way to counteract these overwhelming feelings? The vagus nerve plays a crucial role in this regard.

When you experience stress, your body activates the sympathetic nervous system, also known as the "fight-or-flight" response. This is a primal survival mechanism that prepares your body for immediate action in a perceived threat. Your heart rate increases, breathing becomes shallow, and blood pressure rises.

The vagus nerve, however, acts as a calming counterpoint to this stress response. It's part of the parasympathetic nervous system, often referred to as the "rest-and-digest" system. By stimulating the vagus nerve, you can actively switch off the stress response and promote feelings of peace and well-being. Imagine taking a deep breath and feeling your body instantly relax – that's the power of the vagus nerve in action!

In the next chapter, we'll delve deeper into the science behind vagus nerve stimulation and explore the multitude of benefits you can experience by incorporating simple daily exercises into your routine.

By understanding and activating this powerful nerve, you can unlock a path to a calmer, healthier, and more balanced you.

Chapter 2: Why Daily Vagus Nerve Exercises Matter: Unlocking Your Body's Natural Healing Potential

The vagus nerve isn't just a passive observer in your well-being; it's an active participant with immense potential for healing. This chapter will explore the science behind stimulating the vagus nerve and the many benefits you can reap through daily exercises.

- The Science Behind Vagus Nerve Stimulation

Modern science is increasingly recognizing the power of the vagus nerve. Research is shedding light on the intricate connection between stimulating the vagus nerve and a range of positive health outcomes. Here's a glimpse into the science at play:

Decreased Inflammation: A number of health issues are associated with chronic inflammation. Studies suggest that vagus nerve stimulation can dampen the inflammatory response by influencing the activity of certain immune cells.

Improved Heart Rate Variability: Heart rate variability (HRV) refers to the natural fluctuation in the time between heartbeats. Higher HRV indicates greater adaptability and resilience to stress. Research shows that stimulating the vagus nerve can improve HRV, making you more stress-resistant.

Enhanced Mood and Emotional Regulation: The vagus nerve has a direct connection to the brain regions involved in mood regulation. Studies suggest that stimulating the vagus nerve can positively impact mood, reduce anxiety, and even alleviate symptoms of depression.

- The Benefits of Daily Practice: Reducing Stress, Enhancing Mood, and More

The benefits of incorporating daily vagus nerve exercises into your routine extend far beyond simply feeling calmer. Here's how these exercises can positively impact your life:

Reduced Stress and Anxiety: By activating the "rest-and-digest" response, vagus nerve exercises can effectively counteract the stress response, leading to reduced feelings of anxiety and overall stress levels.

Improved Digestion and Gut Health: The vagus nerve plays a crucial role in gut motility and digestive function. Stimulating the vagus nerve can help regulate digestion, alleviate symptoms of bloating and constipation, and even contribute to a healthier gut microbiome.

Deeper, More Restful Sleep: Trouble sleeping? Vagus nerve stimulation can promote relaxation and prepare your body for restful sleep. By reducing stress and calming the nervous system, you'll be better equipped to drift off to sleep and experience deeper, more restorative sleep cycles.

Enhanced Emotional Regulation: The vagus nerve's connection to brain regions involved in mood regulation can be harnessed through daily exercises. This can lead to improved emotional regulation, helping you manage difficult emotions and fostering a sense of calmness and well-being.

These are just a few of the many ways stimulating the vagus nerve can positively impact your life. Daily exercises are a simple and effective way to unlock this potential and experience a range of health benefits. The next chapter will delve into specific exercises you can incorporate into your daily routine to start reaping the rewards of a happy vagus nerve.

Part 2: Your Personalized 7-Minute Vagus Nerve Exercise Routine

The vagus nerve may be a complex system, but activating its calming influence can be surprisingly simple. This part of the book will equip you with the tools to create your own personalized 7-minute vagus nerve exercise routine. We'll explore core exercises, delve into additional techniques, and guide you on building a sustainable practice for lasting transformation.

Chapter 3: Creating Your Vagus Nerve Sanctuary: Setting the Stage for Success

Before diving into specific exercises, let's create the ideal environment to maximize the benefits. Here's what you'll need to consider:

Environment: Find a quiet, comfortable space free from distractions. Dimming the lights or lighting a calming candle can enhance the atmosphere.

Intention: Approach your practice with a positive intention. Focus on the goal of relaxation and well-being.

Embracing the Daily Practice: Consistency is key! Aim for 7 minutes of daily exercises, ideally at a similar time each day.

Chapter 4: The Core Exercises: Simple Techniques for Powerful Results

This chapter unveils the essential exercises that form the foundation of your 7-minute routine. Remember, consistency is key, so choose exercises you find enjoyable and can easily integrate into your daily life.

Deep Breathing Techniques: Deep, diaphragmatic breathing is a cornerstone of vagus nerve stimulation. Learn proper breathing techniques, such as box breathing or alternate nostril breathing, to activate the relaxation response and promote calmness.

Humming, Chanting, and Gargling: These vocal exercises stimulate the vagus nerve through the vibrations in your vocal cords. Experiment with humming a calming tune, chanting a soothing mantra, or simply gargling with water for designated periods.

Cold Water Exposure: A short burst of cold water exposure can be a powerful tool for resetting your nervous system and activating the vagus nerve. Consider a cold shower splash, a refreshing face wash with cold water, or applying a cold compress to your face for a few seconds.

Acupressure Techniques: Acupressure involves applying gentle pressure to specific points on your body. This chapter will provide a guided approach to acupressure techniques that target specific pathways of the vagus nerve (illustrations will be included for reference).

Chapter 5: Beyond the Basics: Expanding Your Vagus Nerve Toolkit

While the core exercises are a great foundation, there's a whole world of techniques to explore and tailor your routine. This chapter will introduce additional options:

Yoga Postures for Vagus Nerve Health: Specific yoga postures can effectively stimulate the vagus nerve. We'll delve into simple poses that can be incorporated into your routine, with illustrations for guidance.

Mindfulness and Meditation Techniques: Mindfulness practices and meditation can further enhance the calming effects of vagus nerve exercises. Learn simple techniques to quiet your mind and deepen your relaxation.

Exploring Additional Vagus Nerve Stimulation Methods: From applying ice packs to specific areas to incorporating probiotics into your diet, we'll explore other methods to stimulate the vagus nerve and support your overall well-being.

By incorporating a variety of exercises from this section, you can create a personalized and well-rounded 7-minute routine that caters to your preferences and needs.

Chapter 3: Creating Your Vagus Nerve Sanctuary: Setting the Stage for Success

Imagine a haven within your own home, a space dedicated to unlocking the calming power of the vagus nerve. This chapter will guide you on creating your own personalized vagus nerve sanctuary, a quiet corner where you can cultivate relaxation and well-being through daily exercises.

- Environment, Intention, and Embracing the Daily Practice

Environment:

The first step is finding the perfect location. Ideally, this will be a quiet space free from distractions. Close the door, silence notifications on your phone, and let anyone you live with know that this is your dedicated time for relaxation.

Setting the Mood:

Transform your space into a sensory haven. Dim the lights or light some calming candles with soothing scents like lavender or chamomile. Consider playing some

gentle, ambient music or nature sounds to further
enhance the atmosphere.

Comfort is Key:

Choose a comfortable position, either sitting or lying
down. If you're sitting, opt for a chair that offers good
back support. If you prefer lying down, grab a
comfortable yoga mat or a soft blanket. Remember,
you'll be spending just 7 minutes here, so prioritize
comfort that allows you to fully relax.

Intention is Everything:

Before embarking on your exercises, take a moment to
set your intention. Shut your eyes and inhale deeply
many times. Visualize yourself entering a state of calm
and focus on the goal of relaxation and well-being.
Knowing your intention helps your mind and body work
together to achieve the desired outcome.

Embracing the Daily Practice:

Consistency is the magic ingredient for unlocking the
full potential of vagus nerve stimulation. Aim to
dedicate 7 minutes to your daily routine, ideally at a
similar time each day. This consistency helps train your
body to recognize this time as a dedicated period for

relaxation, making it easier to switch on the "rest-and-digest" response.

Think of your vagus nerve sanctuary as a daily investment in your well-being. By creating a comfortable and calming environment, setting your intention, and committing to consistent practice, you'll be well on your way to reaping the rewards of a happy vagus nerve.

- Tailoring Your Routine: Considerations for Individual Needs

While the core exercises outlined in the next chapter provide a solid foundation for your vagus nerve stimulation routine, it's important to personalize your practice to maximize its effectiveness. Here are some key considerations to tailor your routine to your individual needs:

Listen to Your Body:

The beauty of vagus nerve exercises lies in their gentle and adaptable nature. Pay attention to your body's signals and adjust the exercises accordingly. For example, if a particular breathing technique feels uncomfortable, explore another option. Similarly, if cold water exposure feels too intense, try a cooler temperature or a shorter duration.

Addressing Specific Concerns:

Do you struggle with chronic anxiety? Perhaps you have difficulty falling asleep. Consider incorporating additional exercises that cater to your specific concerns. For instance, research suggests that extended exhalations during breathing exercises can be particularly effective for managing anxiety.

Building Gradually:

If you're new to vagus nerve exercises, it's wise to start slow and gradually increase the duration and intensity of your routine. Begin with a few minutes of practice and build up to the full 7 minutes as your comfort level increases. This allows your body to adjust to the new stimuli and prevents potential overwhelm.

Listen to Your Preferences:

Not everyone enjoys the same exercises. Embrace the variety offered in this book and experiment to find what resonates most with you. Do you find humming relaxing? Great! If not, explore other vocal exercises like chanting or gargling. The key is to choose techniques you find enjoyable and are more likely to integrate into your daily practice.

Medical Considerations:

While generally safe for most individuals, it's important to consult with your doctor before starting any new exercise routine, especially if you have any underlying health conditions. Your doctor can advise you on any potential risks or modifications necessary for your specific situation.

Combining Techniques:

The beauty of vagus nerve stimulation lies in its versatility. Don't be afraid to combine different exercises from the core routine and additional options explored in later chapters. For example, you might start with a few minutes of deep breathing, followed by acupressure techniques, and finish with some gentle yoga postures. Find a combination that leaves you feeling relaxed and rejuvenated.

By tailoring your vagus nerve stimulation routine to your individual needs and preferences, you'll create a practice that feels authentic and sustainable. Remember, consistency is key, so choose exercises you enjoy and can easily incorporate into your daily life. The next chapter will unveil the essential core exercises that form the foundation of your personalized 7-minute routine.

Chapter 4: The Core Exercises: Simple Techniques for Powerful Results

Now that you've created your personalized vagus nerve sanctuary, it's time to explore the essential exercises that will form the foundation of your 7-minute routine. Remember, consistency is key, so choose techniques you find enjoyable and can easily integrate into your daily life. Here are the core exercises that will unlock the calming power of the vagus nerve:

1. Deep Breathing Techniques:

Deep, diaphragmatic breathing is a cornerstone of vagus nerve stimulation. Unlike shallow chest breathing, diaphragmatic breathing engages your diaphragm, the large muscle below your lungs. This type of breathing activates the relaxation response, promoting feelings of calmness and reducing stress.

Box Breathing: This simple technique is a great way to slow down your breathing and activate the parasympathetic nervous system. Here's how to do it:

1. Take a slow, four-count breath through your nose.
2. For four counts, hold your breath.

3. Take a leisurely, four-count breath out through your mouth.
4. For four counts, hold your breath.
5. Continue in this manner for a few minutes.

Alternate Nostril Breathing: This technique can help clear your mind and promote relaxation. Here's how to do it:

1. Take a comfortable seat with a straight back.
2. Close your right nostril with your thumb.
3. Inhale slowly through your left nostril.
4. For four counts, hold your breath.
5. Use your ring finger to close your left nostril.
6. Exhale slowly through your right nostril.
7. Repeat steps 3-6, alternating nostrils for several minutes.

2. Humming, Chanting, and Gargling:

These vocal exercises stimulate the vagus nerve through the vibrations in your vocal cords. They can be a fun and effective way to activate the relaxation response and promote feelings of calm.

Humming: Find a comfortable pitch and simply hum a calming tune for several minutes. You can even try humming along to your favorite relaxing music.

Chanting: Chanting a calming mantra, like "Om" or a favorite phrase that resonates with you, can be a powerful tool for focusing your mind and promoting relaxation.

Gargling: Gargling with cool water for 30 seconds to a minute can be a surprisingly effective way to stimulate the vagus nerve. The act of gargling activates the muscles in your throat and sends signals to the vagus nerve.

3. Cold Water Exposure:

A short burst of cold water exposure can be a powerful tool for resetting your nervous system and activating the vagus nerve. The initial shock triggers the "fight-or-flight" response, but your body quickly rebounds and activates the parasympathetic nervous system, promoting relaxation.

Cold Shower Splash: End your warm shower with a quick 30-second blast of cold water.

Refreshing Face Wash: Splash your face with cold water for a few seconds.

Cold Compress: Apply a cold compress to your face or neck for a few seconds.

Remember: Start slow, especially with cold water exposure. If you're new to this technique, begin with a shorter duration or cooler temperature and gradually increase the intensity as you become more comfortable.

These core exercises are a powerful starting point for your vagus nerve stimulation routine.

- Acupressure Techniques: Targeting Specific Vagus Nerve Pathways

The core exercises introduced in the previous chapter provide a solid foundation for your vagus nerve stimulation routine. This section delves deeper into one specific technique: acupressure. Acupressure involves applying gentle pressure to specific points on your body believed to influence energy flow and promote well-being. Here, we'll explore acupressure techniques that target specific pathways of the vagus nerve. Illustrations are included for your reference.

Important Note: While generally safe for most individuals, it's advisable to consult with a licensed acupressure practitioner before applying significant pressure, especially if you have any underlying health conditions.

Acupressure Points for Vagus Nerve Stimulation:

1. Yin Tang (Third Eye Point):

Location: This point is located between your eyebrows, in the indentation above the bridge of your nose. (See Illustration 1)

Technique: Gently apply pressure to this point with your index finger for 30 seconds to 1 minute. You can also slowly massage the area in a circular motion.

2. ST36 (Stomach 36):

Location: This point is located on the outer leg, four finger-widths below your kneecap and one finger-width to the outside of your shinbone. (See Illustration 2) **Technique:** Apply firm pressure to this point with your thumb for 30 seconds to 1 minute. You can also use a rounded tool like a massage stick for added pressure.

3. LV3 (Liver 3):

Location: This point is located on the top of your foot, between the first and second metatarsals (the long bones in the foot) in the webbing between your toes. (See Illustration 3)

Technique: Apply gentle pressure to this point with your thumb for 30 seconds to 1 minute on each foot. You can also gently massage the area in a circular motion.

Additional Tips:

Breathe: Focus on slow, deep breaths while applying acupressure. This will further enhance the relaxation response.

Bilateral Stimulation: When applicable, stimulate acupressure points on both sides of the body for a balanced effect.

Listen to Your Body: Pay attention to your body's signals. If any point feels uncomfortable, ease off the pressure or discontinue stimulation altogether.

By incorporating these acupressure techniques into your routine, you can target specific pathways of the vagus nerve and promote feelings of calm and well-being. The next chapter will explore additional techniques you can integrate into your practice, including yoga postures and mindfulness exercises, to create a well-rounded and personalized 7-minute routine.

Chapter 5: Beyond the Basics: Expanding Your Vagus Nerve Toolkit

The core exercises and acupressure techniques explored in previous chapters provide a powerful foundation for stimulating your vagus nerve. However, the world of vagus nerve stimulation offers a vast array of options you can incorporate to create a well-rounded and personalized 7-minute routine. This chapter delves into additional techniques to expand your vagus nerve toolkit:

1. Yoga Postures for Vagus Nerve Health:

Specific yoga postures can effectively stimulate the vagus nerve by activating the diaphragm, stretching and massaging internal organs, and promoting relaxation. Here are a few simple yoga poses to consider integrating into your routine:

Child's Pose (Balasana): This gentle pose helps quiet the mind and encourages deep breathing, both of which stimulate the vagus nerve. Put your toes together and place your knees hip-width apart on the ground. With your arms out in front of you, take a seat back on your heels and place your forehead on the mat. Take a deep breath and hold it for a few moments.

Downward-Facing Dog (Adho Mukha Svanasana):
This invigorating pose stretches and strengthens the
entire body, including the internal organs. Start on your
hands and knees with your knees hip-width apart and
hands shoulder-width apart. As much as is comfortable,
straighten your legs by pushing your hips back and up.
Keep your heels flat on the floor (or close to it) and gaze
back towards your heels. Hold for several breaths.

Supine Twist (Supta Matsyendrasana): This gentle
twist helps massage the internal organs and stimulates
the vagus nerve. Lie on your back with your arms
extended out to the sides. Bring your right knee up
towards your chest and gently twist your torso to the left,
keeping your right shoulder grounded on the mat. Look
over your left shoulder and hold for several breaths.
Repeat on the other side.

2. Mindfulness and Meditation Techniques:

Mindfulness practices and meditation can further
enhance the calming effects of vagus nerve exercises.
These techniques help quiet the mind, reduce stress
hormones, and promote relaxation, all of which
contribute to vagus nerve stimulation. To get you going,
try these easy exercises:

Body Scan Meditation: Lie down comfortably and close your eyes. Focus your attention on different parts of your body, one at a time. Notice any physical sensations without judgment. As you scan your body, take slow, deep breaths.

Mindful Breathing: Find a quiet place and sit comfortably. Pay attention to your breathing and notice how your chest or abdomen rises and falls with each breath in and out. Refocus your attention on your breathing if your thoughts stray.

Guided Meditation: There are many guided meditations available online or through apps that can help you focus on relaxation and activate the vagus nerve.

3. Exploring Additional Vagus Nerve Stimulation Methods:

Beyond the exercises covered so far, there are other ways to stimulate the vagus nerve and support your overall well-being:

Probiotics: Studies suggest that a healthy gut microbiome can positively influence the vagus nerve. Incorporating probiotics into your diet through fermented foods or supplements may be beneficial.

Singing and Music: Singing activates the vocal cords, sending signals through the vagus nerve. Listening to calming music can also promote relaxation and vagus nerve activity.

Massage: A gentle massage can stimulate the vagus nerve through touch and promote relaxation. Consider self-massage techniques or a professional massage focused on activating the vagus nerve.

Cold Shower: While a cold shower splash is a core exercise, some individuals may find a full cold shower invigorating and stimulating to the vagus nerve.

By incorporating a variety of techniques from this chapter alongside the core exercises, you can create a personalized and well-rounded 7-minute routine that caters to your preferences and needs. Remember, consistency is key! The more you practice, the more you'll experience the calming and stress-reducing benefits of a happy vagus nerve.

Part 3: Integrating Vagus Nerve Exercises for Lasting Transformation

The journey to a calmer, healthier you through vagus nerve stimulation has just begun. Part 3 will equip you with the tools to seamlessly integrate these practices into your daily life and unlock lasting transformation.

Chapter 6: Making Vagus Nerve Exercises a Habit

Building a sustainable practice is key to reaping the long-term benefits of vagus nerve stimulation. This chapter will guide you on establishing habits that make your 7-minute routine an effortless part of your day.

Start Small: Don't overwhelm yourself – begin with just a few minutes of daily practice and gradually increase the duration as it becomes a habit. Consistency is more important than length initially.

Find Your Time: Identify a time in your day that works best for you, whether it's first thing in the morning or before bed. Consistency in timing reinforces the habit loop.

Pair it with Existing Routines: Link your vagus nerve exercises to an existing habit, such as brushing your teeth or making coffee. This association helps solidify the practice in your routine.

Monitor Your Development: It may be inspiring to maintain a basic journal to record your advancement. Note how you feel before and after your exercises, or use a mood tracker app to monitor changes.

Celebrate Your Successes: Acknowledge your commitment to your practice and celebrate your progress, no matter how small. The habit loop is strengthened by this positive reinforcement.

Chapter 7: Vagus Nerve Stimulation Beyond the 7 Minutes

While the 7-minute routine is a potent tool, vagus nerve stimulation can be integrated throughout your day for even greater benefits. This chapter explores ways to weave these practices into your daily life:

Mindful Movement: Incorporate mindful movements throughout your day. Take the stairs instead of the elevator, stretch at your desk, or go for a short walk during your lunch break.

Laughter is the Best Medicine: Laughter is a powerful stress reliever and stimulates the vagus nerve. Make time for activities that bring you joy and laughter, even if it's just a few minutes a day.

Social Connection: Strong social connections are essential for well-being. Spend time with loved ones, engage in meaningful conversations, and nurture your social network. Social interaction stimulates the vagus nerve and promotes feelings of safety and calm.

Gratitude Practice: Taking time to appreciate the good things in your life can significantly impact your well-being. Start a gratitude journal, or simply take a few minutes each day to reflect on what you're grateful for. Gratitude activates the vagus nerve and promotes feelings of positivity.

Mindful Eating: Slow down and savor your meals. Pay attention to your body's hunger cues and stop eating when you're comfortably full. Mindful eating practices stimulate the vagus nerve and support healthy digestion.

Chapter 8: The Road to Lasting Transformation

Vagus nerve stimulation is not a quick fix; it's a journey towards a healthier, calmer you. This chapter explores the long-term benefits you can expect and offers guidance for overcoming challenges.

Reduced Stress and Anxiety: Regular vagus nerve stimulation can significantly reduce chronic stress and anxiety, leading to a more peaceful and balanced life.

Improved Sleep Quality: Stimulating the vagus nerve promotes relaxation and prepares your body for restful sleep.

Enhanced Mood and Emotional Regulation: By calming the nervous system, vagus nerve exercises can improve your mood and emotional well-being.

Boosted Digestion and Gut Health: The vagus nerve plays a crucial role in digestion. Regular stimulation can improve gut motility and support a healthy gut microbiome.

Overall Well-being: By integrating vagus nerve stimulation into your life, you can experience a sense of overall well-being, increased resilience to stress, and a brighter outlook on life.

Challenges and Solutions:

Finding Time: Everyone is busy, but even a few minutes a day can make a difference. Prioritize your well-being and find pockets of time for your practice.

Lack of Motivation: Starting a new habit takes effort. Track your progress, celebrate your successes, and find an accountability partner if needed.

Difficulty Quieting Your Mind: It's normal for your mind to wander during meditation or breathing exercises. Gently redirect your attention and focus on the present moment. With practice, it will become easier.

Conclusion:

By incorporating the simple yet powerful practices outlined in this book, you can unlock the transformative potential of the vagus nerve. With dedication and consistency, you'll be well on your way to a calmer, healthier, and more balanced you. Remember, the journey to well-being is a

Chapter 6: Building Your Daily Practice: Making Vagus Nerve Exercises a Habit

Congratulations on taking the first steps towards a calmer and healthier you! Now comes the crucial part: establishing a sustainable practice to reap the long-term benefits of vagus nerve stimulation. This chapter will equip you with the tools to seamlessly integrate these practices into your daily life, transforming your 7-minute routine into a habit that sticks.

The Power of Habit:

Habits are powerful automated behaviors that become ingrained in our daily routines. Building a vagus nerve stimulation habit requires dedication and consistency, but the rewards are well worth the effort. Here are some key strategies to make your 7-minute practice an effortless part of your day:

Start Small, Dream Big:
Don't overwhelm yourself trying to achieve a lengthy routine right away. Begin with just 2-3 minutes of daily practice. Focus on consistency over duration. As the practice becomes ingrained, gradually increase the length of your routine to reach your ideal 7 minutes.

Find Your Time:
Identify a specific time in your day that works best for you, whether it's first thing in the morning to set the tone for a calm day, or before bed to unwind and prepare for restful sleep. Consistency in timing strengthens the habit loop, reminding your body and mind that it's time for vagus nerve stimulation.

Pair it with Existing Routines:
Weave your vagus nerve exercises into an existing habit you already perform daily. For example, do your deep breathing exercises right after brushing your teeth in the morning, or practice humming while making your coffee. This association helps solidify the practice in your routine and makes it less likely to be forgotten.

Track Your Progress:
Keeping a simple journal can be a powerful motivator. Note how you feel before and after your exercises. Did you experience a decrease in stress? Improved focus? Track your progress over time to witness the positive changes and celebrate your commitment to your well-being. Consider using a mood tracker app to monitor your emotional shifts as you integrate these practices.

Celebrate Your Successes:

Acknowledge your dedication to your practice and celebrate your progress, no matter how small. Did you manage a full 7 minutes today? Great! Did you squeeze in a quick breathing exercise in the middle of a busy day? Even better! Positive reinforcement strengthens the habit loop and keeps you motivated to continue.

- Building a Sustainable Routine

Remember, building a habit takes time and effort. There will be days when you might miss your practice, but don't get discouraged. The important thing is to resume your course as soon as you can. Here are some more pointers for creating a routine that lasts:

Find an Accountability Partner:
Talk to a friend or family member about your objectives and support one another in staying on course. Having someone to hold you accountable can provide extra motivation on challenging days.

Make it Enjoyable:
Choose exercises you find relaxing and enjoyable. If you dislike a particular technique, explore other options and find what resonates most with you. The more you enjoy your practice, the more likely you are to stick with it.

Focus on the Benefits:
Remind yourself of the positive changes you're experiencing, both mentally and physically. Is your sleep improving? Do you feel calmer throughout the day? Focusing on the benefits keeps you motivated and reinforces the value of your practice.

By incorporating these strategies, you can transform your 7-minute routine from a chore into a cherished daily ritual.

- Overcoming Obstacles and Maintaining Your Motivation

Building a vagus nerve stimulation routine is an empowering step towards a healthier you. However, like any new habit, challenges and moments of decreased motivation may arise. This chapter equips you with tools to overcome these hurdles and stay committed to your journey.

Common Challenges and Solutions:

Finding Time: We all lead busy lives. Here's how to make your practice fit:

Break it Down: Instead of viewing it as a monolithic 7 minutes, split your practice into smaller chunks throughout the day. Do 2 minutes of deep breathing in the morning and another 2 minutes before bed.

Prioritize Your Well-being: Think of your practice as an investment in your health, similar to brushing your teeth or eating a nutritious breakfast. Schedule it in your planner and treat it with the importance it deserves.

Identify Hidden Pockets of Time: Can you squeeze in some calming humming while waiting in line for coffee? During a break from work, take a few deep breaths? Look for these hidden pockets of time throughout your day.

Lack of Motivation: It's normal to experience dips in motivation. Here's how to reignite the spark:

Track Your Progress: Keeping a journal or using a mood tracker app helps you visualize your progress. Witnessing the positive changes you're experiencing can be a powerful motivator.

Locate an Accountability Partner: Talk to a friend or relative about your objectives and stay in touch with them on a regular basis. Knowing someone else is on this journey with you can boost your motivation.

Focus on the Benefits: Remind yourself why you started this practice in the first place. Are you feeling less stressed? Sleeping better? Reconnect with the positive changes you're experiencing to reignite your enthusiasm.

Difficulty Quieting Your Mind: Meditation or breathing exercises can be challenging at first. Here are some tips:

Treat yourself with kindness: It's normal for your thoughts to stray. Don't get discouraged – gently redirect your attention back to your breath or mantra.

Start Small: If focusing for extended periods feels overwhelming, begin with shorter meditations and gradually increase the duration as you become more comfortable.

Guided Meditations: Many apps and online resources offer guided meditations that can provide structure and support, especially for beginners.

Staying Motivated for the Long Haul:

Celebrate Your Successes: Give yourself credit for any accomplishments, no matter how tiny. Did you manage a full 7 minutes today? Great! Celebrate every step forward, reinforcing the positive habits you're building.

Make it Enjoyable: Choose exercises you find relaxing and integrate them into activities you already enjoy. Listen to calming music while doing yoga poses, or hum along to your favorite tunes. The more you enjoy your practice, the more likely you are to stick with it.

Focus on the Journey: View your vagus nerve stimulation practice as a lifelong journey, not a destination. There will be ups and downs, but the key is to stay committed and celebrate the progress you make along the way.

The next chapter will explore ways to weave vagus nerve stimulation practices even further into your daily life, maximizing the benefits and creating a lifestyle of well-being.

Chapter 7: The Vagus Nerve and Beyond: A Holistic Approach to Wellbeing

Your 7-minute vagus nerve stimulation routine is a powerful tool, but it's just one piece of the well-being puzzle. This chapter explores how you can integrate vagus nerve stimulation practices into your daily life beyond your dedicated routine, fostering a holistic approach to well-being.

- The Vagus Nerve: A Conductor of Wellbeing

Think of the vagus nerve as the body's "social connector," influencing everything from digestion to mood. By stimulating the vagus nerve, we can promote relaxation, reduce stress, and support overall well-being. However, true well-being encompasses a multifaceted approach. Here are ways to weave vagus nerve awareness into your daily life for a holistic approach:

Mindful Movement: Our bodies are designed to move. Mindful movement practices, like yoga, tai chi, or even mindful walks, not only stimulate the vagus nerve but also improve circulation, reduce stress hormones, and enhance mood.

Laughter is the Best Medicine: Laughter is a powerful stress reliever and activates the vagus nerve. Make time for activities that bring you joy and laughter, even if it's just a few minutes a day with loved ones.

Social Connection: Strong social connections are essential for well-being. Spend quality time with loved ones, engage in meaningful conversations, and nurture your social network. Social interaction stimulates the vagus nerve and promotes feelings of safety and calm.

Nourishing Your Body and Mind:

What we put into our bodies directly impacts our well-being and nervous system function. Here are some dietary and lifestyle practices that support the vagus nerve and promote overall health:

Prioritize a Balanced Diet: A diet rich in fruits, vegetables, whole grains, and lean proteins provides the essential nutrients your body needs to function optimally.

Stay Hydrated: Dehydration can negatively impact your nervous system function. Stay hydrated and promote general health throughout the day by drinking lots of water.

Limit Processed Foods and Added Sugars: Excessive processed foods and added sugars can contribute to inflammation and disrupt gut health, both of which can negatively impact the vagus nerve.

Get Enough Sleep: Chronic sleep deprivation disrupts the nervous system and can impair vagus nerve function. Aim for 7-8 hours of quality sleep each night.

Manage Stress: Chronic stress is detrimental to well-being. Try some healthy stress-reduction techniques, including working out, practicing meditation, or going outside.

- Beyond the Physical: Cultivating a Positive Mindset

Our thoughts and emotions have a profound impact on our physical well-being. Here are some practices that cultivate a positive mindset and support vagus nerve function:

Gratitude Practice: Taking time to appreciate the good things in your life can significantly impact your well-being. Start a gratitude journal, or simply take a few minutes each day to reflect on what you're grateful for. Gratitude activates the vagus nerve and promotes feelings of positivity.

Mindful Eating: Slow down and savor your meals. Pay attention to your body's hunger cues and stop eating when you're comfortably full. Mindful eating practices stimulate the vagus nerve and support healthy digestion.

Mindfulness and Meditation: Regular mindfulness practices and meditation can significantly reduce stress and anxiety, both of which contribute to vagus nerve dysfunction.

By incorporating these practices alongside your dedicated vagus nerve stimulation routine, you'll be well on your way to fostering a holistic approach to well-being.

- Complementary Practices: Nutrition, Sleep, and Exercise for Enhanced Results

Your 7-minute vagus nerve stimulation routine is a powerful foundation for well-being. However, to truly unlock the full potential of vagus nerve health, consider incorporating complementary practices into your lifestyle. This chapter explores the power of nutrition, sleep, and exercise in optimizing your journey.

Nourishing Your Body for Vagus Nerve Health:

The vagus nerve plays a crucial role in digestion and gut health. By adopting a balanced and gut-friendly diet, you can support the vagus nerve and experience even greater well-being. Here are some key dietary considerations:

Prioritize Fiber: Fiber is essential for promoting healthy gut bacteria, which have a positive influence on the vagus nerve. Consume a diet rich in fruits, vegetables, and whole grains.

Choose Prebiotics and Probiotics: Prebiotics act as food for beneficial gut bacteria, while probiotics directly introduce these helpful microbes into your gut. Consider incorporating prebiotic-rich foods like onions, garlic, and asparagus, or explore probiotic supplements after consulting with your doctor.

Limit Processed Foods and Added Sugars: Excessive processed foods and added sugars can disrupt the gut microbiome and contribute to inflammation, both of which can negatively impact the vagus nerve. When possible, choose entire, unprocessed meals.

Stay Hydrated: Dehydration can impair digestion and nervous system function. To stay hydrated and promote general health, make it a goal to sip on lots of water throughout the day.

Sleep: The Foundation for Vagus Nerve Function

Chronic sleep deprivation disrupts the nervous system and can impair vagus nerve function. These pointers can help you give good sleep top priority:

Create a Regular Sleep Schedule: Even on weekends, go to bed and wake up at the same time every day. This aids in maintaining the normal sleep-wake cycle of your body.

Create a Relaxing Bedtime Routine: Develop a calming bedtime routine that helps you unwind before sleep. Read a book, take a warm bath, or engage in relaxation exercises like meditation or deep breathing.

Optimize Your Sleep Environment: Ensure your bedroom is dark, quiet, and cool. Invest in blackout curtains, an earplug mask, and comfortable bedding to create an environment conducive to restful sleep.

Limit Your Screen Time Before Bed: The blue light that electronics emit can interfere with your sleep cycle. Give yourself at least an hour before bed to avoid using screens.

Exercise: A Powerful Ally for Vagus Nerve Health

Regular exercise is not only essential for physical health but also promotes vagus nerve function and overall well-being. Here are some exercise tips for vagus nerve stimulation:

Engage in Activities You Enjoy: Choose physical activities you find enjoyable, whether it's dancing, swimming, brisk walking, or playing a sport. You're more likely to stick with an exercise routine if you find it fun.

Focus on Movement Throughout the Day: Don't limit exercise to dedicated workout sessions. Take the stairs instead of the elevator, stretch at your desk, or go for a short walk during your lunch break.

Incorporate Deep Breathing Exercises: Deep breathing exercises like diaphragmatic breathing activate the vagus nerve and promote relaxation. You can integrate these exercises into your workout routine or practice them throughout the day.

Explore Yoga and Tai Chi: These mindful movement practices combine gentle movements with deep breathing, making them excellent options for vagus nerve stimulation and overall stress reduction.

By incorporating these complementary practices into your lifestyle alongside your vagus nerve stimulation routine, you'll be well on your way to optimizing your well-being. The next chapter will explore the long-term benefits you can expect from this journey and offer guidance for navigating any challenges that may arise.

Chapter 8: The Power Within: The Vagus Nerve as Your Gateway to a Healthier, Happier You

Congratulations! You've embarked on a transformative journey to unlock the power of your vagus nerve. This remarkable nerve, often referred to as the body's "social connector," holds immense potential for enhancing your well-being. By incorporating the practices explored in this book, you've taken a significant step towards a healthier, happier you.

The Long-Term Rewards of Vagus Nerve Stimulation:

By consistently stimulating your vagus nerve, you can expect a multitude of long-term benefits, including:

Reduced Stress and Anxiety: Regular vagus nerve stimulation practices can significantly reduce chronic stress and anxiety, leading to a calmer and more peaceful life.

Improved Sleep Quality: Stimulating the vagus nerve promotes relaxation and prepares your body for restful sleep. You may experience deeper sleep patterns and wake feeling more refreshed.

Enhanced Mood and Emotional Regulation: By calming the nervous system, vagus nerve exercises can improve your mood, emotional resilience, and overall emotional well-being.

Boosted Digestion and Gut Health: The vagus nerve plays a crucial role in digestion. Regular stimulation can improve gut motility, support a healthy gut microbiome, and contribute to a healthier digestive system.

Overall Well-being: By integrating vagus nerve stimulation into your life, you can experience a sense of overall well-being, increased resilience to stress, and a brighter outlook on life.

The vagus nerve is a powerful tool for promoting not only physical health but also mental and emotional well-being. As you continue your practice, you may also experience:

Improved Cognitive Function: Studies suggest that vagus nerve stimulation may enhance cognitive function, memory, and focus.

Decreased Inflammation: A number of medical disorders are associated with chronic inflammation. Vagus nerve stimulation may help reduce inflammation throughout the body.

Stronger Immune System: A healthy vagus nerve may contribute to a more robust immune system, better equipped to fight off illness.

Remember, this is a journey, not a destination. There will be days when you might miss your practice, or challenges may arise. The key is to be kind to yourself, gently get back on track, and celebrate your progress, no matter how small.

Embrace the Power Within:

The vagus nerve is an undeniable force within you, a powerful tool waiting to be harnessed. By integrating the practices in this book and cultivating a holistic approach to well-being, you can unlock the transformative potential of the vagus nerve and empower yourself to live a healthier, happier, and more fulfilling life.

This concludes our exploration of the vagus nerve and its potential for enhancing your well-being. Remember, the power to create a healthier, happier you lies within. Embrace the journey, and may your vagus nerve guide you towards a life filled with peace, vitality, and joy.

Bonus Section

Appendix A: Resources for Further Exploration (Books, Websites, and Research)

Your exploration of the vagus nerve has just begun! This appendix offers resources to deepen your understanding and stay up-to-date on the latest research:

Books:
   * "The Body Keeps the Score" by Bessel van der Kolk
   * "The Vagus Nerve: Healing the Body, Mind, and Soul" by Stanley Rosenberg
   * "Daring Greatly: How the Courage to Be Vulnerable Transforms the Way We Live, Love, Parent, and Lead" by Brené Brown (for fostering a growth mindset and emotional well-being)

Websites:
   * The National Institutes of Health (NIH) offers reliable information on the nervous system, including the vagus nerve: [National Institutes of Health (.gov)](https://www.nih.gov/)

   * The American Psychological Association (APA) provides resources on stress management and relaxation techniques: (https://www.apa.org/)

* The Mayo Clinic has a page dedicated to vagus nerve stimulation: (https://www.mayoclinic.org/tests-procedures/vagus-nerve-stimulation/multimedia/vagus-nerve-stimulation/img-20006852)

Research:

* You can access scholarly articles on the vagus nerve through online databases like PubMed or ScienceDirect. These resources require a library subscription or fee, but some libraries offer free public access.

Appendix B: Troubleshooting Common Challenges and FAQs

Q: I miss my practice sometimes. How can I stay consistent?

A: Building a habit takes time. Be kind to yourself and gently get back on track when you miss a session. Start with shorter practices if needed, and gradually increase the duration as you regain consistency.

Q: I find it difficult to quiet my mind during meditation.

A: It's common to have wandering thoughts. Don't get discouraged – gently redirect your attention back to your breath or mantra. Begin with shorter meditations and gradually increase the duration as you become more comfortable.

Q: I don't experience immediate results. Should I give up?

A: The vagus nerve takes time to respond. Be patient and consistent with your practice. Track your progress in a journal to witness the positive changes over time.

Q: Are there any risks associated with vagus nerve
stimulation exercises?

A: Vagus nerve stimulation exercises are generally
safe for most people. However, if you have any
underlying health conditions, consult with your doctor
before starting any new practices.

Q: Can I do too much vagus nerve stimulation?

A: While there isn't a set limit, listen to your body. If
you experience any discomfort, ease off or stop the
exercise.

This appendix provides a starting point for
troubleshooting common challenges and frequently
asked questions. Remember, consulting a healthcare
professional is always recommended for personalized
guidance.

By incorporating the resources and information in this
bonus section, you can continue your exploration of the
vagus nerve and embark on a lifelong journey towards a
healthier, happier you.